WHEN HUGE IS NOT ENOUGH II

TABLE OF CONTENTS

Disclaimer: before starting any exercise routine or nutritional advice in this book, please consult your Physician.

INTRODUCTION

"When Huge Is Not Enough Part II", will show you the reader what I have learned in the last 30 years since writing the first edition. This new book will build upon what I have done and what I have learned since then. In this book, I will pour my heart out and reveal to you, information that you will never see in any magazine. I will show you brutally advanced and shocking techniques to spur you on to the next level. I will hold nothing back. I will go into excruciating detail. I want everyone to get as big as they want, without ever having to endanger their health from drug use.

I will show you, how at the age of 50, I went from 255lbs to 283 lbs., fast, and naturally of course. I am not interested in fake drug bloated unhealthy muscle. I am not interested in building muscle that I cannot keep. I want you and I to live a long and healthy life of being BRUTALY HUGE!

WHOLE BODY WORKOUT

I was in college for 6 years full time in the 1990's. I graduated in 1995 with a Doctor of Pharmacy degree. I was carrying a full load of 18-21 credits a semester. My priorities changed. I didn't have the time to live in the gym or live the bodybuilding lifestyle. Quite frankly, who would want to be in the gym 6 days a week? I could never understand that? I hate to say it, but a lot of bodybuilding routines have their basis in ignorance.

This section is really for advanced trainers, who are huge, but want to get even bigger than they thought possible, without resorting to the illegal and unsafe use of drugs. I really don't want to waste a lot of time re-hashing the pitfalls of overtraining and recuperation. I would strongly suggest you get the first two books: How to Get Brutally Huge and The Bodyparts.

At any rate I digress. I was in college, studying 10 hours a day, I was in 5 classes every day and didn't have the time to be in the gym. So, I started doing a whole body workout once every 7 days. I did it on Friday night, so I would have the whole weekend off, which was spent working or studying and I had 7 days to recuperate. At this time, I was in my early thirties and believe it or not, my recuperation was already a little slower than in my mid-twenties. Working a muscle once every 7 days fit the bill for recovery and even some growth.

The whole body workouts are great for super busy people. I would focus on the Compound movements that involved working lots of muscles simultaneously. Remember, my focus was on maintaining, not living the bodybuilding lifestyle, while in school, and I even grew somewhat.

Did you know that working three exercises can work almost 80 percent of your body? For example. Doing the following three exercise will do just that. If all you did was squats, rows, and bench press, you would work most of your body.

I remember going to the university campus gym and doing the following workout. Sure, I changed squats for leg presses at times, but the outline remained essentially the same for 6 years.

Example full body routine:

Squats or leg presses–3 to 4 sets
Lat pulldowns or bent rows-3 sets each
Bench press or dips-3 sets each
Lateral raises or shoulder presses-2 sets
Shrugs-2 sets
Weighted good mornings or hyperextensions-2 sets
Calf raises-2 sets

Abdominals-2 sets
Forearms-2 sets

This routine was really good for staying big, while going to school full time and working part time. As school got more difficult, and I was getting older, I noticed problems.

In my last year of school while working on my dissertation, doing 40-50 hours a week of internship, I was always getting sniffles, and run down. Too much intensity and always pushing it was starting to wear me down.

I didn't know it then, but if your goal is to maintain, and you have school, work, and family obligations or lots of stress in your life, then scale back the intensity some. Don't always go to failure on every set, every single workout. As I wrote about in my first books, too much high intensity can fry your nerves, immune system, and recuperation. You need to cycle intensity. Over three workouts, do the first one well short of failure on your exercises, then on the next workout go almost to failure on all your exercises, then on the third workout you can go to extreme failure on the last set of each exercise. This cycling of intensity will keep you growing, and you won't get the sniffles and colds all the time. Looking back, another approach would've been for me to pick two bodyparts I wanted to grow, and just maintain the rest. I point all this out to help you keep working out and not getting sick.

I'm grateful I got through all those years. After I took my board exam, I sort of just quit, and didn't workout for 49 days straight, I remember. I offer this section on full body workouts with the intention of trying to keep you in the game, keep you healthy, and you not getting run down and sick.

If you try this approach, namely full body workouts, cut it down to a bare minimum, be sure you are eating high quality food, sleep 8 hours a night, take naps when you need to, and take a potent multivitamin/mineral tablet daily. Also consider taking what they used to call stress tabs that have a lot of vitamin C, B-complex, and zinc, in one tablet. Or, you can take those separately.

The full body workouts are great and can be very productive. You can free up a lot of time and can even grow if you do it intelligently with proper adherence to rest, supplementation, and nutrition. One of the reasons full body workouts are so productive, is that you are working out so infrequently. However, they will overtrain you if done 2-3 times a week. Stick to once every 5-7 days and you will put on size and weight rapidly. You may really like them.

THE CRO-MAGNON WORKOUT

This may sound like a joke, but there is a reason I call this workout the cro-magnon workout. Cro-magnon's were very brutal and rugged in their build. They were crude, primitive, and, well, they didn't care about cuts or refinement. I've read scholarly articles by paleontologists who have suggested that these people and the Neanderthals were probably 5'8" and weighed 250lbs. One article said they probably looked like weightlifters. They were heavily muscled.

The cro-magnon workout was something I did when I was 29 during college. I was in a community college, worked part time, and could train like a maniac and live the lifestyle of training, eating, and sleeping a lot.

I called the workout the cro-magnon workout because it was brutal, crude, and primitive compared to our sophisticated modern-day bodybuilding routines. Most people are afraid to try this because they have been so brainwashed by the magazines that say you must work every single muscle in your body with 20 sets or be in the gym 4-6 days a week.

If you are stuck in a rut, are a skinny hard gainer, or want a quick spurt of massive growth, then this workout is for you. It is beautiful in its simplicity, but is tortuous in nature, will pack on slabs of brutal muscle fast. At the time, having 20 inch plus arms is all that mattered to me. I didn't care about tie-ins, shape, veins on my belly or trophies. Although if you get a 20 inch arm, you'll have plenty of shape. I thought, when my arms were 24 inches, then I'd worry about cuts. I didn't get overweight by normal societal standards, as my abdominals were still barely showing. I just wanted to lift heavy weights and grow.

All I would do is 3 exercises designed to hit the largest muscles and pack on mass. Sometimes I may have added 1 set each of abs, calves, and lateral raises for maintenance. Here is all that I would do:

1) Squats-135 x 10, 225 x 8, 335 x 6, then 455 x 4reps
2) Dips bodyweight x 15 reps, 70lbs on a dip belt x 6-8 reps, then 135lbs x 3-4 reps.
3) Bent Rows- 135 x 15 reps, 250 x 6 reps, then 365 x 4 reps.

This workout helped me get bigger than I ever was before. For this workout to work, I followed the following principles:

1) Always add weight every workout.
2) Go to complete failure on the last set.

3) I did it once every 5 to 9 days.
4) Eat a lot of food.
5) Do the repetitions slowly and deliberately.
6) Sleep a lot and take naps if needed.

This workout worked because you are doing such a small volume of sets, but because you are resting so long between workout, you couldn't stop yourself from growing. By resting so long, you are absolutely assured of not working out too soon and thus preventing growth from occurring. Warning: if you have a slow metabolism, you may find yourself putting on weight too fast and may need to cut back on the calories or take a 15 minute walk three times a week. If you have a fast metabolism, this routine done once a week will be prefect for you to rest, conserve energy and to gain size and weight. As a matter of fact, if you have a fast metabolism, you may want to cut back on all other sports and physical activities until you put on 20-30 pounds. As far as cardio goes, anyone who has done squats or back work to failure, knows how hard it works your heart and lungs. Most people who do not pace themselves, usually find themselves breathing so heavily they cannot talk after a properly done set of rows or squats. If you can talk after a set, you did not do it hard enough. So, cutting back on other superfluous activities is only short term endeavor until you are 20 lbs. heavier.

People always ask me the following question. When is it time to return to the gym and do the next workout? The answer is simple. Do not ever go back until you feel thick. I don't care what these stupid man-made routines in the magazines say. Just because your soreness is gone from one workout, does not mean you grew. You will feel it when you grow. You'll have this thick, well rounded feeling to your muscles. You'll feel energetic, stronger than ever, and your muscles will feel powerful and all coiled up and ready to explode in the next workout. If you don't feel that way, then you should wait until you do. As mentioned above, not being sore anymore only means you've repaired most of the damage from the previous workout. In other words, your muscles have healed and are back to the size they were before the workout. For growth to occur, it takes even more days of rest after you have repaired yourself. If you are going to do this brutal, gut busting, back breaking workout, you must eat and rest long enough for growth to occur. Depending on your age, size, recuperative abilities, and stress levels in your life, you may need to do this once every 5-9 days. Perhaps resting 5 days if you're young and have a 17-inch arm, maybe resting 9 days, yes 9 days, that's not a typo, especially if you are 30 or 40 years old, with a 19.5-inch arm.

I made some excellent gains on this short but brutal whole body workout. Remember though, you must rest a long time in between workouts. You WILL NOT grow if you do this workout two to three times a week. Summing it up, do this infrequently, go to failure on the last set, add weight or more reps every workout, eat a lot, sleep a lot, and you WILL experience great gains doing this routine. You will always feel thick and powerful too. Lastly, feeling so thick will make you feel good psychologically speaking and you will feel good about yourself.

SLOW MOTION TRAINING

I did not invent slow motion training. However, I am going to show you how I incorporated slow motion training into my system to help me get some of the best gains in quality muscle, density, and size that I have ever achieved in my life. As a matter of fact, it will be hard to stop yourself from growing if you do it right. Slow Motion training and Super Slow Motion training helped propel me from 255lbs up to 283lbs in a few years. Furthermore, I accomplished this at the age of 50.

Slow motion training is where you might take 10 seconds to move a weight up, pause a second, then take 10 seconds to lower the weight. There is no bouncing at the bottom of any rep on any exercise, and on any exercise where you could lock out, you don't. You keep the muscle under full tension for the whole repetition and indeed, the whole set. Super slow motion training is where you might take 15-20 seconds to move a weight up, then 15-20 seconds to lower it. Again, there is never any bouncing or locking out. All the reps are started off very slowly, deliberately, and with full control. Also, you deliberately tense the muscle all throughout the range of motion. It's kind of like isometrics, but in in slow motion.

This first benefit of slow motion training that I would like to tell you about is that of increased cardiovascular and cardiorespiratory conditioning. If you go to the cable pulldown machine, use an underhand grip, and take 10 seconds to pull it down and 10 seconds to let it up, you will immediately notice a few things. First, you won't be able to breathe too well. Second, you will start feeling uncomfortable and sweating profusely. Third, you'll see your arms quivering and shaking right in front of you. Lastly, it will burn so badly, that I'm afraid some of you won't be able to take the pain and quit. Trust me, it's easier to cheat curl 200lbs, because your biceps don't feel anything, as momentum, and your lower back are doing all the work, and not your biceps. If you persist, you will get better at this tortuous manner of slow motion training.

The second benefit I noticed after months of training in this fashion, was that of the muscles getting harder and denser. As we get bigger, we must find more ways of increasing the intensity to induce further gains. This is especially true if you are a natural trainer. Slow motion training is brutal, and it focuses the intensity on the muscle and causes searing pain like no other training method I have ever tried.

Third, with slow motion training, I started growing again. Even low sets and resting long periods in between workouts wasn't inducing further gains. Slow motion training is so shockingly brutal, it will stimulate grow in ways you never imagined were possible.

Fourth, you will not be able to train in the usual sloppy form some lifters do, namely deadlifting 500lbs, screaming, jerking the weight up, and then crashing it on the floor to prove how strong they are. The fact that you can't train as heavy, but that you use moderate weights in complete control, is a blessing on your joints. When you are always in control, moving the weight slowly, never bouncing, jerking, or locking out, your joints never hurt, and it's almost impossible to get hurt.

Lastly, you'll build lasting gains. I have noticed that when I take layoffs, I never lose anything, as a matter of fact, I gain a couple of pounds and grow. The muscles get so dense and thick, that I would have to take a month off to even start to feel soft.

Despite all the benefits, here's the reason so many of you won't be able handle this kind of training. For one, some people cannot mentally handle lifting anything but heavy weights. They must always show off in the gym. Their egos will not permit them to bench press 200 lbs. when they were bouncing 300lbs off their chest. Two, since slow motion training is more intense than anything you can imagine, you'll require even more rest time to grow. The first few times you do slow motion training to failure, you will be raw the next day. You might be sore two or three days as a matter of fact. Thirdly, some of you will be lacking in faith to try something so radically different. Once you decide to start slow motion training, do not rest for the same amount of time between workouts that you did before starting this type of training. You must rest even more, or you simply won't grow. But a lot of you won't be able to handle this fact because you're so afraid to trust and of losing your precious little gains. I understand wanting to work out, but I want to grow more! I expect and demand some kind gains to show for it.

Let me tell you one thing that'll happen when training like this. You'll be on the bench press, doing your reps, 10 seconds up, 10 seconds down, no locking out, pause at the bottom for 1 second before starting the next rep up. Some helpful, but uninformed person will run up to save you, thinking you are so weak that you are getting stuck, pull the bar off you, and then ask you what were you doing. It has really happened to me. It's infuriating. Usually if I see someone's hands get near my bar, I bark out an order and say don't help me!!! Some people's egos can't handle benching 225lbs when they used to do 315lbs. That's so sad because they'll never know what kind of gains they're missing out on. You'll get weird looks at first, like what are you doing. Some people are so worried about what others think. I only care about one thing and that's getting results. The last reason that I can see most people not getting this correctly is that of not being able to stand staying out of the gym and resting even more days. Look, do you want a 19 or 20 inch arm or not?

When I was making the best gains of my life at 50, I was working a bodypart once every 10 days. Working out once every ten days was to grow by the way, and not just maintain. I cannot stress this enough times, how important it is, that you undo this bodybuilding brainwashing you have experienced from reading the magazines. You absolutely must get rid of this stupid concept of the week based on 7 days. Where I reside, there is no "week". You rest as long as it takes to feel thick, and then you do it again. That is the greatest pearl I can ever give you. So many bodybuilders can't mentally accept this fact. I don't waste time trying to convince anyone anymore. With most people, their attitude is, if you didn't win a contest, you don't know anything, even if you're like me and have arms that are 19 inches hanging at the side. I'm going to say it again, to get huge, get rid of the notion of the 7-day week. Time was invented by people to keep track of things and get a schedule to life. Your recuperative powers don't obey the 7 day week. They don't adhere to the concept of a 7 day week. It will take as long as it takes to recover and feel thick. You have got to thoroughly embrace this, or you will never get BRUTALLY HUGE, and you MUST allow your body to heal and do its thing in its own time. You must get rid of the concept of the 7 day week. This last paragraph could literally mean the difference of you getting a 17 inch vs 19 inch arm. You will know when you are doing this right when you always feel thick and rested. Please, give this a few weeks. You can always go back to your erroneous ways of training.

When I was 50, here is the way I trained. First of all, and to rebel against the conventionally accepted bodybuilding wisdom, I quit doing the staid leg/back/bicep and chest/shoulder/triceps workout in favor of doing upper body one day and lower body the other day split.

So, here are my two workouts:
Workout A-Upper body
Workout B-lower body
W/O is an abbreviation for workout

I would do each workout for the same muscles on the tenth day. See chart below:

Day	Mon	Tue	Wed	Thu	Fri	Sat	Sun	Mon	Tue	Wed
w/o	A	Rest	rest	rest	Rest	B	Rest	Rest	Rest	rest

On the tenth day, I'd repeat the above sequence. I can't begin to tell you how thick I felt. Why did I rest 10 days you ask, because empirical evidence taught me that was how long it took for me to rest, grow and feel thick all over. One of the reasons, I do the whole upper body in one workout is that it is difficult to separate the muscles as so many of them are inter-related. For example, when you do pullovers, they work your pecs, lats, and rear triceps. If you haven't noticed that, you're doing them wrong. So, do you put them on back or chest day? Shoulders are involved in almost everything, including chest and back. I did this on every tenth day, because on day 4 I was still sore, on day 7 I was not sore, but felt flat, and by day 9 or 10, I felt thick as a brick. In short, I learned to work with my recuperative powers and wait as long as it took to feel thick! That is the greatest gift I can ever give you. It is one you will never see mentioned in a magazine. Ask yourself this: what do the champs know about natural training? Not much in my opinion.

Next is the actual routine I'd follow to grow and get thicker than ever. I prefer to do compound movements and don't even like isolation movements for arms, as there is no amount of weight you can do in curls, that works your arms like 350lb rows to failure. Also, doing rows to failure, for example, will stimulate your whole body and metabolism, whereas curls wont. Below is my typical split:

<u>Upper Body</u>:
Close grip bench presses-2 sets, 4-6 then 3 reps
One arm Rows- 2 sets, 6 reps, then 3-4 reps
Shrugs- 2 sets, 6 reps, then 4 reps
Weighted Good mornings- 2 sets, 6 reps then 4.
One arm laterals- 2 sets, 10 reps, then 6 reps
Wrist curls-2 sets, 10 reps, then 6 reps
Reverse Wrist curls-2 sets, 10 reps, then 6 reps

<u>Lower Body</u>:
Leg Presses: 3 sets of 10,6,4 reps
Standing Calves-2 sets of 10,6 reps
Tibialis raises- 1 set of 10-20 reps
Abs-1 set of 20 reps

If you'll notice, there is an extremely low number of reps being done here. With slow motion training, you must do away with the concept of the number of reps being done. Your new focus should be that of how long you stress the muscle. Two repetitions taking 1 total minute to perform is more stressful then 6 sloppy reps done in 15 seconds. What's critical here is to go to failure, and you will, regardless of the number of reps. I'd be willing to bet, that most of you who can bench press 300lbs, would find your arms quivering and begging for mercy from benching 185lbs for a 20 second rep, with no lockout to give you a rest, and holding at the bottom for one second before deliberately and under full control pressing the weight back up.

While we are on the subject of reps, lets make sure you thoroughly understand how to do a rep properly with slow motion training. The goal is to stress the muscle more than you ever have in your life. Indeed, as you get bigger, you must find ways of putting more and more focused stress on the muscle than you ever have before. It's sort of a law of diminishing returns, trying harder and harder, while seemingly getting less and less. However, the irony here, is that as you give more and more effort, coupled with longer rests in between workouts, you will get back more and more growth. At this stage, as you may have surmised, the cheating principle is out! It is not intense enough. Too many other muscles end up doing the work intended for the targeted muscle.

So, let us explore how to do a rep properly, so as to get the feeling of maximal thickness in a few days to a week. We'll use the close grip bench press as an example of one exercise that will hit the pecs, front delts, and triceps. Believe it or not, because your elbows travel up and down farther, this will work your pecs harder than imagined.

Lay down on your bench on a Smith Machine. From a high position, unlock the weight, take 10 seconds to slowly lower the bar. Purposely tense the triceps harder than you need to while remaining in full control of the weight as you lower it. At the bottom, hold it about ¼ of an inch off your chest for 2 seconds. You do not want to rest at the bottom. Very deliberately start tensing the pecs and triceps until the weight ever so slowly starts to move upwards. As you get to the top, repeat this process and try to get 3-4 reps, if you can. This is so hard you can't believe it. Each repetition is taking about 25-30 seconds! There are two main goals here: 1) never give the muscle a rest, and 2) always remain in full control. There is never to be an explosive initiation of the reps. You MUST super slowly initiate and move the weight an agonizing quarter of an inch at a time. To ensure you are taking about 10 seconds to go up, you can count to yourself, 1001,1002,1003, and so on, up to ten seconds.

This kind of training is so intense, you must keep the sets down to about 2-3 sets total. You do not want to do 3 sets for chest and 2-3 for triceps. You have just done all you'll ever need to do. Remember, it's not about having a "good workout", which is usually a euphemism for overtraining, it's about how can you annihilate a muscle with the least amount of sets. I know some of you probably won't be able to handle this. This is sad, because this I what real training is about, and it's exactly what you need to get explosive, healthy, and lasting gains. No one said it was going to be easy.

We are now going to look at another exercise and see how I used slow motion training as a way to get phenomenal leg development, as well as stimulate my whole metabolism and to help produce gains over the whole body.

The exercise we will explore is the leg press. I really like leg presses as a way to get massive thighs. Here is how I combined slow motion, continuous tension, progressive weight overload, long rests between workouts, and training to failure as a way to get Brutally Huge.

When I did leg presses, I'd release the supports and take ten seconds to lower the weight. Then I would pause at the bottom for 1-2 seconds. I do not go all the way down where the weight is pushing your thighs into your chest and you are in essence just relaxing. I stop a little short of that point. I keep tension on the thigh. I also stop because, I don't wont any kind of bounce, or momentum to help. Also, you never want to reverse direction on a dime. After the 1-2 second pause at the bottom, I start building pressure, tensing the thigh harder and harder, before the weight even starts to move. Once it does start to move, you want it to be done with great deliberation, no explosiveness, and very slowly. You should be in agony training like this. Now the weight should take about 10 seconds to ever so slowly get back up to the top. However, we don't to lock out as that would be resting. We want to stop the weight about 2-3 inches of your knees locking out. Near the top, you will now pause 1-2 seconds, holding the weight up there, keeping tension on the thighs, before deliberately and slowly letting the weight go back down for another exhausting rep. Remember, we are not concerned with the notion of doing a certain number of reps any more. Just one of these reps, 20 seconds in all, or 40 seconds with super slow could replace a traditional set of 6-10 reps. In short, your thighs will be suffering throughout the whole set and never get a rest, even if that set is only 2-4 reps. Lastly, when using slow motion training, you want to use the heaviest you can for 2-4 repetitions. It's not an excuse to train lightly.

Below is an example of how my leg press workout looked. Remember, one exercise per body part, preferably compound movements, are all you will ever need. Forget the silly nonsense about needing 4-5 exercises so you work all areas of the thigh. If you do one exercise properly, as outlined above, the workout will annihilate all the fibers in the thigh, as you get closer to failure, hidden fibers will be recruited to try and help out and they too will get worked hard. Remember, having a "good workout", doing 20 sets, is a euphemism for overtraining. So again, here is the leg press workout, with the best weights I ever handled in the slow motion manner of training:

Leg Press=225 x 10, 500 x 8, 875 x 4 reps.

As a warmup, I'd do 15 minutes on the exercise cycle, to get some cardio, and to warm up the knees. Then, I'd proceed with the above demonstrated leg press workout. One thing I want to give you, to increase your longevity of your knee joints is this. On squats or leg presses, the sudden torque of reversing direction on a dime, can be really hard on the medial aspect, or inside of your knee joint (vs the lateral aspect or outside of the knee joint). If you are experiencing twinges of pain on the inside of your knee joint, slow motion training can help alleviate that. Knees can be hurt by jarring movements, impact, grinding, and over use. As mentioned above, when doing leg presses, just lower the sled to where your lower leg is at a 90 degree angle to your thigh. Do not worry about doing full reps. They are not intense enough to stimulate growth and can hurt your joints. Besides, your thighs resting on your chest is a rest. We do not want the muscle resting! Instead, when you are "at the bottom", with your lower leg at 90 degree angle to your thigh, we want you to hold the weight suspended in mid air for 1-2 seconds, now while holding, start tensing the thigh harder and harder until it starts to move. Resist the urge to "hurry it up" because it hurts. Actually, the speed of the repetition should be the slowest when first starting to move the weight upwards. Going super slow at the start is what will help stop the pain in the knee joint. Also, at the top, never lockout because not only are you resting there, but bone is grinding on bone! If you do not listen to me, you might be hearing it from an orthopedic surgeon in 10-20 years.

Lastly, be sure to rest long periods of time between workouts. Rest longer than you used to. Remember, you MUST get rid of this notion of your week being based on a Monday through Sunday routine. For most people, depending on your life's stresses, age, and size, 6 to 10 days of rest between bodyparts should be enough. Be sure to add weight every workout, even if it's only 5 lbs. How strong you are mentally will also determine how big you get. Can you take this kind of agony? You must resist the urge to escape the pain, to make it easy on yourself. If you can, new gains await you.

Lastly, while this book is meant only for advanced trainers, I feel that I better give a quick idea of what your workout schedule should look like. If you will notice, there will be a progression of how long you rest as you get bigger. There will also be a progression of how long you rest as you get older or are more stressed out.

Assuming the traditional leg/back/bicep and chest/shoulder/triceps split, here is how often you should be working out. Remember, this is a good approximation, and we will assume you are about 5'10" and have an 18 inch arm. Remember, this is not written in stone. A 17" arm at 5'6" is just as advanced as a 18 inch arm at 5'10" and a 19 inch arm at 6'1" is advanced. If you are a beginner or intermediate trainer, please consult my other books "How to Get Brutally Huge" and "The Bodyparts". Again, these suggested routines are for people who are fairly huge and are stuck in their progress.

Workout A- legs/back/biceps
Workout B- chest/shoulders/ triceps
W/O = workout

If you are a teenager, with 18 inch arms, who can recuperate fast, the following schedule will allow you enough rest to row. In essence, you will be working each body part about once every 6th day.

Day	Mon	Tues	Wed	Thu	Fri	Sat	Sun
Workout	A	Rest	Rest	B	Rest	rest	A

If you are in your twenties and have an 18 inch arm, you need to rest a little longer. I would recommend working a body part once every 7 days. Before you laugh, remember world class powerlifters, who weigh 300lbs, only do squats, deadlifts, and bench presses once a week.

Day	Mon	Tue	Wed	Thu	Fri	Sat	Sun	Mon
W/O	A	Rest	Rest	Rest	B	Rest	Rest	A

If you are in your thirties, things are "slowing down", compared to being 16 years old. You may be working 40 or more hours a week and are stressed out. Below is the schedule I would recommend for more growth, assuming you are already large. I would recommend working a body part once every 8th day.

Day	Mon	Tue	Wed	Thu	Fri	Sat	Sun	Mon	Tue
W/O	A	Rest	Rest	Rest	B	Rest	Rest	Rest	A

If you are in your forties, and you have an 18 inch arm, or you are 5'6" with a 17 inch arm for example, you should probably workout about once every 9th day or so. Below is how the schedule, not "week" should look.

Day	Mon	Tue	Wed	Thu	Fri	Sat	Sun	Mon	Tue	Wed
w/o	A	Off	Off	Off	B	Off	Off	Off	Off	A

If you are in your fifties like me, and want to really grow still, then you probably need to consider working out once every 10th day. Remember what I said earlier, you will never hear this stuff from any magazine. What do they know?

Day	Mon	Tue	Wed	Thu	Fri	Sat	Sun	Mon	Tue	Wed
w/o	A	off	off	off	off	B	Off	Off	Off	off

I am now 59 years young! I optimally like to train a body part once every 11 days to achieve growth and can do once every 14-17 days just to maintain! Remember as you get bigger, older, or more stressed out, or are generating incredibly stress and intensity in each workout, you need to rest more in order to grow.

In closing, I believe that if you apply the slow motion principle, in the way I have outlined in this chapter, you will experience incredible gains, even if you are already large, and especially if you have never trained in this fashion before. Good luck and get ready to make some of the best gains you have ever experienced.

SLOW MOTION DEADLIFTS

In this chapter, you will see how I periodically used deadlifts to help me go from 255 to 283lbs in a few years, at the age of 50. This chapter is going to blow away everything you ever thought you knew about the proper way to do deadlifts. For one, you will not be concerned about trying to show off in the gym, lifting "5 plates", bellowing, screaming, and smashing the weight on the floor to show everyone how manly you are. You will be using this exercise to stimulate overall body mass, build incredible back thickness, and stimulate your metabolism towards further size and weight gains.

First, load up your bar with a warmup weight. Squat down and grab the bar. You can use the traditional one hand over, one hand under grip on the bar. Now, kind of slightly hyperextend your back without moving the bar. Lift your head up slightly. Start tensing every muscle in your body. The weight has still not started moving. Now slowly start lifting the weight off the floor. You want to take about ten seconds to raise up to a position that is about 6 inches short of standing erect or locking out. When you think you are at that near top position, pull your elbows backwards, toward your sides, all the while supporting that weight in midair, about 6 inches short of standing erect. You will feel your lats contract hard. At the same time, while suspended in mid air, slightly arch your back upwards to contract your erectors even harder. At this point, your erectors, lats, and inner back should all be forcefully contracted. Hold the contraction a couple of seconds before slowly lowering the bar to the floor. Do not let it drop or smash the floor. Unlike the pause in the leg press reps near the bottom of the rep, when the weight is at the floor, the bar should touch the floor so softly that no one even hears it. It will be a "gentle" touch and go. It's almost as if the bar didn't even touch the floor. Do it this way so your thighs and back muscles don't get one second of rest. Also, forget about that silly leaning way back at the top of the movement. You will never get that far. You do not need to lean back like that. That is just an excuse to rest. This movement when done properly, will be a cross between a deadlift where you squat down and mostly use your thighs, and a stiff leg deadlift, which is mostly the back, but again, you will slightly bend your knees, grab the bar, look up, tense all the back muscles, then deliberately initiate the 10 second rep. Your back should never be rounded forward.

When I did deadlifts in this manner, my back started feeling so thick, that I couldn't believe it. My entire back was exploding with new found thickness. Also, to save time, at the end of each deadlift set, I may stand there and shrug the bar in slow motion for 4-6 reps. Consider it a sort of a time saving super set so I didn't have to do shrugs separately, wasting time, and over training the traps by working them twice. Yes, the traps get worked very hard from deadlifts, and you don't want to do them separately again, on a different day, when doing shoulders or something.

One last thing, when doing a deadlift in super slow motion, don't be surprised if your thighs pump up. Furthermore, it will be okay to eliminate direct thigh work as this manner of doing deadlifts will work them sufficiently enough to at least maintain them if not grow a little. You'll know if you're over training your thighs by doing deadlifts and direct work, as your thighs will start feeling small, and you'll start feeling burned out. Another warning is, you will most likely not need to do any direct lat work when you do these deadlifts as described above, as there will be an intense contraction of the lats if done properly. If you try doing lat pulls or rows in conjunction with the slow motion deadlifts, you will probably over train your erectors and or lats. Please trust me on this. It's always better to do too little than to do too much and not grow.

Below is a sample deadlift workout I did. You will not need or be able to lift a lot when training in this fashion. You will also be quite out of breath if you do these in the manner described above. Talk about "back breaking work".

Example deadlift workout:
Deadlifts- 135 x 6, 205 x 4, 295 x 3-4 reps

I mentioned above that when you do deadlifts this way, you may not want to, or need to do direct leg work, rows, or lat pulls.

So, I would kind of revert back to the old leg/back /bicep/ forearms split.

My workout looked like this:
Deadlifts/shrugs- 3 sets of 6,4,4 reps.
Barbell curls-2 sets 6,4 reps
Wrist curls-2 sets
Reverse wrist curls-1 set

Then on the other workout I would do chest/ shoulders/and triceps.

In conclusion, start doing your deadlifts as described above, notice how your overall metabolism is stimulated, you'll always be hungry, therefore eat more, gain weight, and explode to new levels of growth and size.

ROW SLOW FOR HUGE BICEPS

In this chapter, you the reader will learn my secrets for getting BRUTALLY HUGE biceps without doing any curls. As a matter of fact, if you did try to do direct bicep work after doing rows in the way I will shortly show you, you would grotesquely over train your biceps, they will feel small, not grow, and maybe even shrink. You have got to get over your unrealistic fear of losing size if you do not do enough or as much as you think you should. Doing enough is always about doing too many sets. It rarely is ever not overtraining. Trust me, one slow super intense rep will at the very least maintain your size. With slow motion training, you will feel it more, and get more growth out of one 20 second rep, than you would from three conventionally done sets. By conventional, I mean the way most people ignorantly do their sets which is to heave the weight up and down, in sloppy form, just to get the set done and impress their buddies.

So, without much fanfare, let us get down to the mechanics of how to do a row, combined with slow motion, in a way that will make your biceps explode. I have determined that 2 sets are all you will need. One of the advantages of slow motion training, is that since it is done so slowly, and since you are always in control, it is hard to get hurt. You can do a 3rd set with light weights if you wish, as a warmup, before hitting the 2 sets that count.

First, after a light set of rows (which I don't do), grab a weight that is about 55-60% of your max weight. If you are rowing with on arm, you can rest the opposite knee and hand on a bench. With your arm hanging at your side, ever so slowly, and with deliberation, start pulling the weight up towards your chest. It should take about 10 seconds for the dumbbell to touch your chest. You'll notice your bicep quivering and shaking as you do this. That is good! That is a sign you are doing it correctly. At the top, hold it against your torso for anywhere from 4-10 seconds for a peak contraction effect that you'll feel in your lats. Remember, I am showing you how to do your rows in a fashion that'll make your biceps explode, but we don't want to ignore your lats and inner back either. Also, doing a peak contraction at the top for your lats will help exhaust them so that the biceps have to work even harder as the lats will be too exhausted to help. Now slowly lower the weight back towards the beginning area but stop slightly short of letting the weight dangle with your arm out straight, as that'll let your bicep relax. We do not want the bicep relaxing. If you are only going to do 2 sets, you really must make every rep count. Do the first set for about 6 reps. You should be almost fatigued to the point of failure.

You can stop here, or go to failure, and you will experience better growth. On the second or last set, you will want to go to failure.

You do not want to run from the pain! In no way do you want to make this easy on yourself. You want to do everything you can to make it harder. That's why this shocks you into such incredible spurts of growth. If done properly, when you flex your biceps, they should feel jammed full of blood, thick, and tight.

Here are a few additional principles to follow. Add weight or do an extra rep whenever possible. I feel you will never need to worry about sets of ten reps again. Two to four reps of slow motion will be more intense, more brutal, and produce more gains than a bunch of sets done in the traditional manner. You never want to bounce the weights up and down, like with some kind of rhythm. You do not want any kind of tempo. Your reps all need to be initiated deliberately and with full control. Be sure not to add in any direct bicep work. Lastly, for me at my stage, I have found that you should change the exercise after every 3rd workout, to really shake things up. I have noticed the first workout of a new exercise is hard and you feel awkward. The second time, it's easier and you can handle some more weight, and perform it easier. For me, by the 3rd workout, my biceps are kind of getting used to it, and after that, I don't gain much. In other words, I start plateauing after the 3rd workout. Again, I mention ten seconds as the time you should use to go up and ten seconds to lower the weight, but find the time that it takes to make your biceps quiver in agony, make your forehead perspire, your breathing is difficult, and the rep is so painful to even perform. You might need 8 seconds, 10 seconds, or 15 seconds to get the desired effect. The bottom line is slow it down enough to where your biceps are working excruciatingly hard.

Some of my favorite exercises, that I like to do in a manner conducive towards biceps growth are one arm DB rows, Bent barbell rows, Seated cable rows, Close reverse grip pulldowns, and Underhand cable pulldowns. Below is a typical one arm DB row workout that I do.

One arm DB rows. Example workout below:

One arm rows- 80lbs x 6reps, 140lbs x 4 reps.

This may not seem like a lot. Granted, it isn't. That's the whole point. There is no way you can over train if all you do is two sets! However, the slow motion reps focus the intensity on a muscle in much the same way a magnifying glass can focus sunlight on a piece of wood and burn it. Your biceps will feel this. Now, as long as you wait about 6-10 days between workouts, you will grow. It's really that simple, yet so brutally hard. That's why it works.

In conclusion, if you really want baseball sized biceps, please give the above techniques a try and don't add more sets. If you do, then don't blame me if you don't grow. More is never better, unless it is more rest, more days between workouts, more weight, and more laser like focus and intensity on each rep. Each and every rep should be more intense than one whole set done in the traditional manner. Resist the urge to cheat. Do not run from the pain but do everything in your power to make the set more deliberate and difficult. If you follow these principles, you will get the massive arms you have always desired.

FOR BRUTAL ARMS STOP WORKING THEM

What I am about to share with you, I discovered by serendipity. It was a combination of factors that led me to this revolutionary way of training. I think I have mentioned this before, but it was 1994 and I was in college. I decided for the first time in my life, to train to failure on my underhand lat machine pulldowns. I only did 2 sets. I went to failure on both sets. On the warmup set with 180lbs, I slowly did about 15 reps. Then on the second and last set with about 220lbs, I slowly and strictly did about 4 reps. There was no jerking, or fast movements. They were very controlled. This may seem like not very heavy weights, but for all my college years, I was pretty much maintaining, and doing full body workouts. I was also running 45 minutes a week in the sandy washes here in Tucson, but I digress, that is another story.

I was like everyone else. I did my back first, then did biceps after them. I used the typical pyramid scheme, warming up on a succession of sets while pacing myself. The first time I did back work to failure, my biceps exploded from the shock of this type of training. They looked visibly bigger and when I measured them, they were ¼ inch bigger from just that one workout.

The other fact that led me to even try this type of training, quite honestly was disgust with the results of my biceps training. I hadn't grown in years and was fed up doing direct biceps work or curls. I figured, well, my arms aren't growing anyway, why work them. I'll just do heavy back work to failure and maintain them. Why do anymore than I have to, I thought to myself. Sorry to disappoint all of you, but I do not want to be in the gym for 2 hours just for the heck of it, or if I will not grow from it.

Well, this new founded way of training started me on a road to discovery, which ultimately led me to some of the best gains in my life. I wasn't growing nonstop, but for the first time in my life my arms always felt thick. It wouldn't be until many more years that I stumbled upon the concept of slow motion training. It was then, that I had a combination that started building really thick massive arms. Someone I knew once commented that my arms looked like legs.

So now we will get into some routines you can do, that'll blast your arms, and believe it or not, build torso size if you give it all you've got. You can pick 2 exercises, a pushing movement and a pulling movement. So, if some of you are frustrated with your arm progress, give these sample routines a try and do not add extra sets.

Routine 1
Close grip Benches- 135 x 4, 185 x 4, 235 x 4
1 arm DB rows- 80 x 8 reps, 140 x 4 reps

The above workout will train your pecs, front delts, with an emphasis on triceps, and will work your lats, biceps and brachioradialis. I would do all the reps over 20 seconds, that is, 10 seconds up, hold, then 10 seconds down. With the hold and pause at top added in, the reps were probably 25 seconds long. So, a set of 4 reps took almost 2 full minutes. The last set of course would be to failure, I'd add weight every workout, and I'd rest 9 days between workouts. I'm not a naturally strong person and the most weight I ever handled this strictly in the one arm rows was 160lb dumbbells and in the close grips, about 255lbs. I also admit to having done 3 sets on the close grips, as the elbows and shoulders can be delicate, and you want to warm them up thoroughly. Sometimes, I'd change from a power routine and do two sets to failure.

Close grip Benches-135 x 12, then 205lbs x 6
One arm rows- 85 x 10, 125lb x 6

On the above 135 x 12 close grips, you may laugh at going to failure with such a pathetically light weight, but remember, the time to do that one set was 12 x 25 seconds, or about 3 minutes. Think about that, my triceps and pecs were in searing pain for 3 whole minutes. They did not hurt, if at all, when I used to do 6 sloppy reps as done by most people. You have t mentally get over "only using" 225lbs when you used to bounce 300lbs. Slow motion reps with 225lbs feels like 300lbs. Lastly, after exhausting my triceps like that, I couldn't handle the usual 235lb x 4, so I had to drop the weight. The pump you will achieve will be phenomenal. I like using the Smith machine for presses as you do not need a spotter. If you use free weights, consider getting someone to spot you. Explain to them what you are doing so they will be patient and not grab the bar and help you just because they think you are getting stuck because you appear to be going slowly and struggling. Also, with free weights, if your triceps go numb and the weight drops, you will be glad you have a spotter.

Here is another sample arm workout, that'll also explode your back and chest:

Bent over Rows-135 x 10 then 225 x 6
Incline barbell Press-135 x6,185 x 4, 225 x 3-4

I want to emphasize, that if you want to place maximal stress and focus on making your biceps grow from back work, then you want to concentrate on the first 8 inches of any rowing or pulling movement. So, when you start your one arm rows for example, really look at your biceps, watch them quiver, and focus on the initial part of the movement, striving to go exceptionally slow in this portion of the movement. With your bent rows, it is better to look ahead, rather than at your biceps, so as to keep your back straight. It is this extreme difficulty and irritation you will feel, that will give you the growth you have only dreamed of. Here is an experiment to prove the point. Find a chinning bar. Hang from it for 30-60 seconds. Using a reverse grip, hands about 10 inches apart, pull up only 2 inches and hold the whole time if you can. When you let go and drop to the ground, flex your biceps, you should notice quite a pump. More importantly, you got it at the beginning of the rep, and from sustained stress on the muscle. This should prove something to you. Use the same thinking when doing pressing movements for your triceps.

Lastly, I would like to show you how you can use shoulder pressing movements to blast your triceps and deltoids. No longer will you need separate triceps movements.

My favorite is the standing front press with a barbell. I only do two sets. With the bar on a rack about face level, I get under the bar, with a fairly close grip, and my hands are maybe 15 inches apart. I step back and slowly, over 10 seconds deliberately press the weight up. I stop a few inches short of locking out. Remember, at this stage, we never want to rest during a single rep, or at any point in a set. After holding the weight at the top for 4-8 seconds, I take ten seconds to lower the weight. You can lower the weight all the way down but keep the triceps and deltoids tensed. In other words, you are working to hold the weight about 1 inch short of true bottom, or just resting on your upper chest. Now I do the second set. To really make the triceps and deltoids really scream, I slowly, over ten seconds press the weight up, hold at the top for 4-8 seconds, but now only lower the bar to about chin level, hold a few seconds, then start pressing up, and repeat the sequence until exhausted.

When you use shoulder pressing movements to work your triceps and deltoids, DO NOT do the 2-3 sets of close grip bench presses or any chest pressing movement as you will then be doing 4-5 sets of super intense triceps work and that will over train them. When I am doing shoulder pressing movements to work the triceps, you may be asking, well, what do I do for the pectoral muscles then?

What I use is the pec dec and perform 2 sets to work the chest. With slow motion on the warmup set, there is no need to do 5 sets of an exercise to get safely warmed up. Again, you are going so slow it is difficult to get hurt and, you are going to failure on the warmup. The pump you will get will be incredible. But we are getting off track here. Below is the workout I use to make my triceps grow, using shoulder pressing movements, in a way that will also grow your deltoids, and at the very least maintain your pectoral mass with the Pec Decs.

Standing Overhead Press-warmup, then 115lbs x 6 reps, then 155lbs x 4 reps.

You may be asking, why the emphasis on triceps? The answer is simple. It is hard to get a 20 inch arm by only working your biceps. Anatomically speaking, two thirds of your arm mass are triceps. If you want that arm to look HUGE just hanging there and if you want to stretch that tape to 20 inches, you must over develop the triceps, especially the rear head.

Give the above principles a try and your arms will achieve new levels of growth you never thought possible. But remember, if you do not increase the rest time between workouts, do not blame me if your arms don't grow.

THE PITFALLS OF 4 DAY A WEEK TRAINING AND HIGH INTENSITY ROUTINES

Many bodybuilders use the 4 days a week routine, which is a lot better than 6 days a week. I kind of touched on this earlier, but I want to show you why this type of training will limit your gains. I am not theorizing here. I actually had my gains screech to a halt at 19 years of age training like this. I was doing the usual: Leg/Back/Biceps on Monday and Thursday Chest/Shoulders/ Triceps on Tuesday and Friday. How nifty, it even rhymes.

I was starting to feel chronically fatigued all over. The constant heavy training to failure and not resting long enough was getting to me. I ached everywhere and did not want to work out. There comes a time where you are big enough and you maybe training so intensely that 3 days of rest is not enough. This really irritates me! Who said it is enough? What are their credentials? Did some magazine say so? What does any drug bloated bodybuilder know about the art and science of natural recuperation vs "forced growth" at all costs? I am asking you to think. I am asking you to listen to what your body is telling you.

When you are big, an arm that size, training to maximal intensity and failure, causes so much damage, and stress on your recuperative systems, that there is no way you can totally recover and grow on top of it, in 3 short days. Then to add further insult, after Monday's workout, you are working out again on Tuesday!!! I know, I know, you are working different muscles you say, right? So, the muscles you worked on Monday's workout are resting right? Wrong! I have said this in my previous books that all the energy you are wasting working out again on Tuesday, could've been directed towards healing the muscles you worked out on Monday. This is the biggest reason most of you get Stuck at 17-18 inches while using the 4 day a week training routine. I'm going to cut to the chase. The only big people who can grow resting so little, are the one's taking lots of drugs. Trust me, you do not want to go that route! A natural trainee can never recuperate that fast. Recuperation takes longer when you are natural! You will know I'm right about this if your muscles feel achy, small, flat, and you feel kind of lethargic and you really don't want to go to the gym using the 4 day a week training methodology.

The whole purpose of this book is to give natural trainers an alternative to the use of unsafe, illegal, and dangerous drugs that will hurt you or end your life prematurely. I would strongly suggest you get a copy of one of my other books, How to Get Brutally Huge, to understand recuperation and how long you should rest between workouts. This is an advanced book for advanced lifters, but I will give a quick glimpse into how often you should be training to rest enough to grow.

If your arms are about 17 inches, the 4 day a week routine will work. If they are up to 18 inches, you may want to consider resting 4-5 days between workouts. If your arms are 19 inches, you may need to rest 6 days between workouts. For each decade you get older, add an extra day of rest on top of that. Now you know why, at 59, I work out once every 10th day. I am growing too. You must learn to work with your body, rest, and you will grow again. I know this is going to be a very difficult concept to accept, mostly because the bodybuilding magazines wont ever tell you this. If you only knew how wrong everything you read in those magazines is, for you the natural trainer. I will repeat it again, you cannot grow naturally, doing those drug based routines. If you try to, you will just stay stuck at your current levels, feel small, run down, sickly, and eventually probably give up in frustration.

DIET AND SUPPLEMENTS

A lot of people have asked me how to eat to grow. I confess, I have not always talked about nutrition in prior books. There is really nothing mysterious about it. If you are losing weight, you are not eating enough. If you are getting fat, you are eating too much. Find a balance where you always feel thick, not starved or small. You should never feel hungry when you are trying to grow. A good starting point is 30 calories per kilogram. Depending on your age and metabolism, you may need more or less.

When we are young, we can do a lot wrong nutritionally and grow. When I was young and single, I thought a ½ lb. of pasta, with tomato sauce and a quart of milk was a good diet. I was really wrong. However, I grew back then!

Below I will give you some sample meals. For protein, I like to consume about one gram of protein per kilogram of weight. So, if you weigh 220lbs, which is 100 kilograms of weight, you could eat 100 grams of protein. Additionally, if you have any kidney problems, you may need less and always drink enough water each day to make sure you are hydrated and flush your kidneys properly. In Arizona, when it's 115 degrees outside, we can easily drink a gallon when outside, and if working outside, or working out hard, we may need 1-2 gallons of fluids, while in the heat. It depends also on where you live. For carbohydrates I try to shun sugar and simple carbs in favor of healthy complex carbs. Examples of such would be brown rice, green leafy vegetables, mixed vegetables, and baked potatoes. Fats are so important. I know the conventional wisdom out there says they are bad, but you need sufficient amounts of dietary fat for your nerves, skin, hair, joints, and overall health. The only bad fats I know of are trans fats like those found in donuts! Even saturated fats like butter are good for you, and are safer to eat than margarine. Decades ago, a noted famous trainer said, when you train naturally, you must gain 1 lb. of fat for every 3 pounds of muscle that you gain. If you think you can get ripped, stay that way, and grow naturally, you are seriously misguided. Did you know that every nerve in your body is covered by a phospholipid sheath? I do not believe in all these supplements, that bodybuilding ads claim will make you look like a champ, but only waste your money.

Below is a sample culinary day in my life. Warning, occasionally, I love a pizza or a bowl of ice cream. I'm sorry, but I want to enjoy life, not be neurotic about a vein on my belly.

Meal one (pre breakfast)- a very small bowl of oatmeal, raisons, organic brown cane sugar with collagen powder added in (collagen is good for the joints).

Meal two breakfast 2)- A blender bottle with 8 oz organic raw milk, 6 ounces coffee, 1 scoop (20 grams of protein) of whey protein powder, 1 teaspoon of Stevia or organic cane sugar and vanilla extract for taste. I may add one raw egg from cage free hens. They're superior in nutrition and taste. When you cook one, you will notice the yolk is orange, vs pale yellow from a "traditional" egg.

Meal three (lunch)-A turkey, avocado, bacon, and spinach sandwich with a lot of filtered water. Or, alternatively, I may have a peanut butter with honey sandwich with 4 oz of milk.

Meal four (dinner)- ½ pound salmon, brown or wild rice, and broccoli or zucchinis and squash. Maybe I'll have a beer too.

Snack before bed- 4 oz. organic raw milk, and a few cashews, or a hard-boiled egg.

You can eat what you want. Sometimes dinner is pot roast, spaghetti, turkey breast, or chicken. I rarely eat pasta anymore, unless it's made from organic wheat or ancient grains. I only eat ancient grain bread. When I was 18, I could eat 8-11 thousand calories daily when I had a fast metabolism. Now, 40 years later, I may consume 3-5 thousand calories daily, and my weight is stable and steady. After most meals, I will have a piece of pineapple to help aid in digestion. Pineapple has bromelain which helps aid in digestion, and therefore, absorbing more of what you eat. If a meal is particularly big, I may have an enzyme tablet (with lipase, protease, amylase, and other enzymes added in it) or a bromelain tablet. You'll be surprised how flat your belly feels after using one of these, even with a big meal. I never eat seconds at this point, as I do not wish to ever weigh 300lbs. I'm currently 278lbs, and that's enough. But if you're underweight, young, have a fast metabolism, or your job is such that you need the additional calories, then by all means, do so.

Below is a list of supplements I use and why I use them.

Multimineral/vitamin- Everyone should take one daily. These days, your diet may be deficient in vitamins and minerals especially if you eat lots of fast food, which you should not.
Vitamin C -I take 2grams in the AM and 2 grams in the PM. For adrenal health, recuperation, and immunity.
B Complex- 1 cap twice daily for nervous health and energy metabolism.
Ginger (1 piece) or Ginseng. These are called adaptogens, and can help your adrenal health, especially if you feel run down.

Glucosamine, chondroitin, MSM, and gelatin- these are good for the cartilage in your joints, and the joints themselves. Start taking them when you are young, so when you are old, your joints do not bother you.

Magnesium capsule- one daily for adrenal health. High intensity training can really overwork your adrenal system.

Fish oil capsules- I like salmon fish oil capsules. I like to take a few a day, as the omega fatty acids can be beneficial for your joints, and brain. I'm over 50, so to ensure good eye health, I take a lutein capsule every day with zeaxanthin.

Of particular importance, I always use sea salt. Regular table salt has only sodium chloride, and small amounts of iodine. The composition varies, and you can look this up, but various sea salts have roughly 80 minerals in them. Also, if you have high blood pressure, a lot of doctors recommend it over table salt. There is potassium, magnesium, and manganese in sea salt, which can cause vasodilation of the blood vessels and a reduction in blood pressure. Furthermore, I feel it tastes better.

I confess I really like dark chocolate. Dark chocolate, unlike milk chocolate, contains antioxidants, stimulants, and bioflavonoids. The bioflavonoids can cause arterial vasodilation and subsequent reduction in blood pressure. It tastes good and can lift your mood too. Beyond these supplements, I do not believe in a whole lot of other bodybuilding supplements that "suggest" or claim will make you look like Mr Olympia. I feel you would be better off spending your money on good food. I do believe in basic supplements to stay healthy. That's pretty much it in my typical nutritional day.

CONCLUSION

It has been a little over 30 years since I wrote When Huge is Not Enough. In that time, I have learned a lot. There are times when I had other priorities in life, but I never stopped working out and trying to learn new and more powerful techniques to propel me to new levels of development. I must admit that a lot my discoveries happened as the result of being frustrated and fed up with no gains. Some of my newer discoveries where found by continually searching for some new knowledge.

To summarize everything that has been covered in this book, as you get bigger, you must find ever more intense methods of stimulating growth and you will need more and more time to rest. Resting is what allows you to grow. Training is only the stimulus. Performing too many sets or engaging in training too frequently is what keeps most trainers from ever getting HUGE. Resting more and more will work wonders, but only up to a point. Trying to get stronger will only get you so far. There comes a time when we must find ever more brutal ways of training to increase the stress on a muscle. We must find ways to focus more direct stress on a muscle. We must place greater demands on a muscle without overtraining it. We must do less sets but do them more intensely than ever before. Overtraining, as you are well aware of by now, is the enemy of growth.

As the amount of focused stress on a muscle increases, the more damage there is done to the muscles, your nerves, and your recovery systems. That is why I advocate longer and longer periods of rest as you get bigger, or want to get bigger, and are older, or you are under lots of stress.

In this book, we have combined the principles of undertraining, progressive overload, eating enough to grow, increasing the intensity, putting more stress on the muscle, and taking longer recuperation periods than ever before, so as to allow grow to occur. This would especially be true if you are older, working full time, and have other stressful demands in life, whether it be family or careers.

I cannot stress it enough; growth will only occur if you stimulate a muscle with ever more stressful demands and then back off and let the muscle rest so that growth can occur. I firmly believe that if you practice the principles outlined in this book, you will experience some of the best gains in your life, even if you are 35, 45, or 50 like I was when all of this came together for me. I feel like I was rewarded for a lifetime of dedicating myself to natural bodybuilding. For me the best really did come near the end.

Please do not ever resort to taking the horrible drugs that a lot of bodybuilders take. They are illegal and they will hurt your health. You cannot abuse your body like that for 10,20, 30 years and expect to have a lifetime of good health. You do not want to go down that path. It is not worth it. Trust me, at 40, you will not care about your plastic Mr. Podunk trophy that you won by using drugs when you were 20. The plastic trophy will not matter to you when you are 45 and plagued with health problems and you are now small and weak. You will be happier to be both healthy and Huge. Ignore me at your own discretion and peril.

Dedicate yourself to mastering the principles contained in this book, and you too can be Brutally Huge and live a long life. There is no reason you cannot have your cake and eat it too. You can be Huge until your 60's, 70's, maybe even 80's. I will let you know when I get there. I'm 59 now and I'm still Brutally Huge, train harder than when I was 20, and still enjoying some of the best gains of my life.

God bless you, best wishes, stay healthy and get Brutally HUGE!